HOME REMEDIES FOR <u>CHILD</u> BEDWETTING

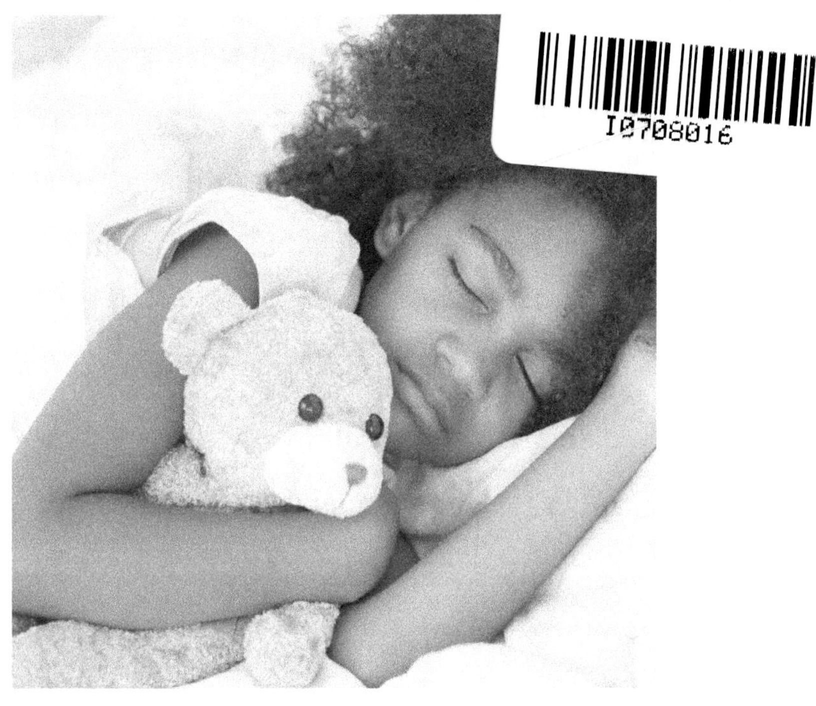

Safe and Effective Natural Solutions
for a Better Night's Sleep

James L. Prince

Copyright

All rights reserved. No part of this publication may be reproduced, distributed, or transmitted in any form or by any means, including photocopying, recording, or other electronic or mechanical methods, without the prior written permission of the publisher, except in the case of brief quotations embodied in critical reviews and certain other noncommercial uses permitted by copyright law.

Table of content

FOREWORD

As a parent, I know firsthand how difficult it can be to address the issue of child bedwetting. It can be a source of stress, confusion and embarrassment for both parent and child. I am thrilled to be writing the foreword for this book which provides an in-depth look at the topic of child bedwetting.

This book dives into the causes of bedwetting, treatment options, and tips for both parents and children.

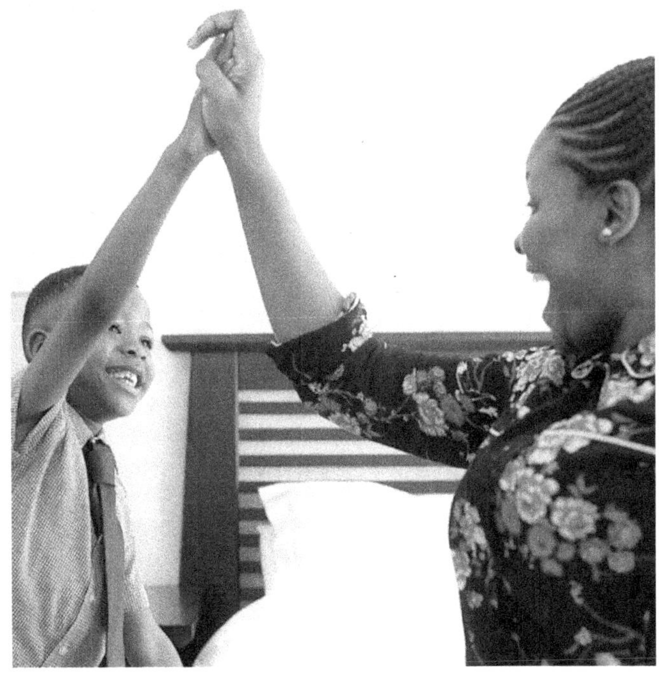

It also looks at the emotional and psychological impacts of bedwetting, as well as how to cope with the stress and anxiety it can cause. It is full of useful advice that parents can use to help their children overcome bedwetting and move on with their lives.

I believe this book is a must-read for anyone who is dealing with the issue of child bedwetting. It is a comprehensive and accessible resource that will help parents understand the issue and provide their children with the support they need.

I hope that this book will provide the guidance and support that parents and children need to tackle this difficult issue.

Introduction

Child bedwetting is a common problem that affects many children. It is also called nocturnal enuresis and is defined as the involuntary release of urine during sleep. It is estimated that 15% of 5-year-olds still wet the bed and that 5 to 7 million children in the United States are affected. Boys are more prone to bedwetting than females are.

It can be a source of embarrassment and frustration for children and their parents.

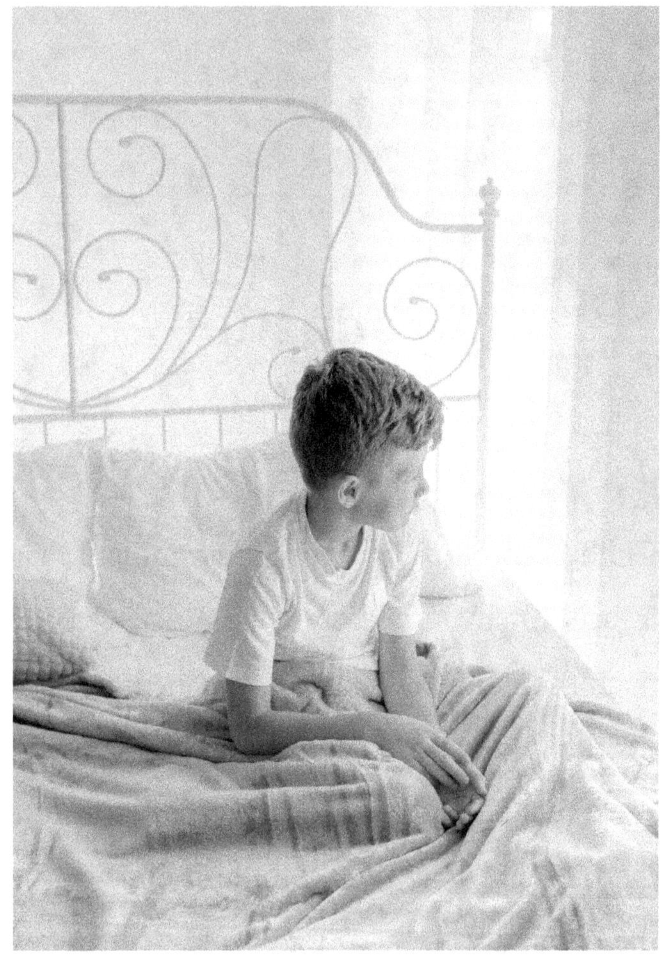

However, it is important to remember that most children will outgrow this problem with time. It is also important to understand that bedwetting is not the child's fault and that it is not caused by emotional or psychological problems. Treatment options include lifestyle changes, medications, and psychological therapies.

If your child is bedwetting, it is important to talk to your paediatrician. They can provide you with knowledge and tools to support your child. Remember, bedwetting is a very common problem and most children will outgrow it.

Chapter 1

Bedwetting in Children

Children frequently have nocturnal enuresis, sometimes known as bedwetting. It is estimated that 5-7 million children in the United States wet the bed at least once a week. Bedwetting can be caused by a variety of factors, such as medical issues, hormonal imbalances, environmental factors, or even psychological problems.

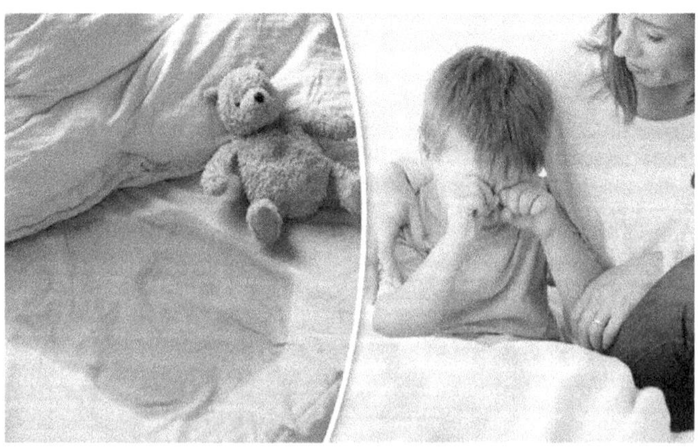

There are several treatments available for bedwetting in children. The most common approaches are behavioural treatments, such as scheduled toilet visits, and medical treatments, such as medications and bedwetting alarms. Behavioural treatments involve teaching the child to recognize the signals that indicate they need to use the toilet and to respond quickly to these signals.

Medical treatments involve taking medications that reduce the amount of urine produced at night, or using bedwetting alarms that alert the child when they have wet the bed.

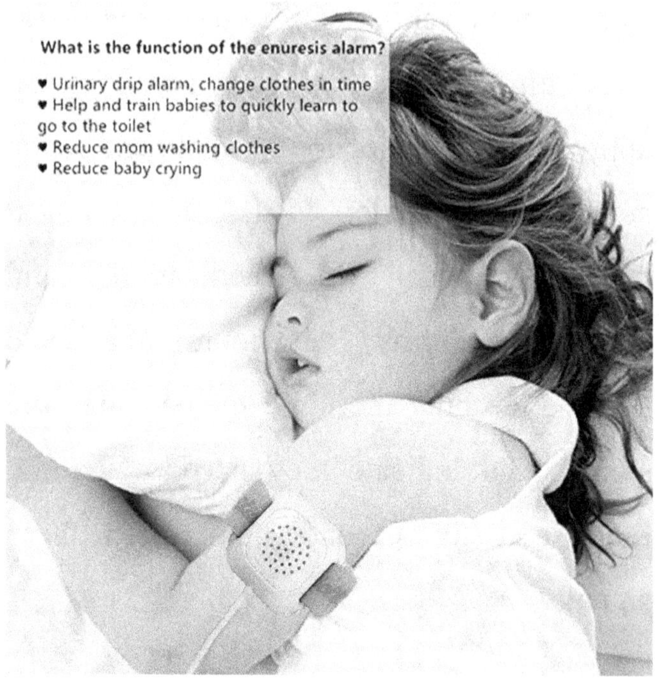

Parents should also work with their children to ensure they are drinking enough fluids during the day and avoiding beverages that contain caffeine or alcohol in the evening. Additionally, parents should ensure their children are getting enough sleep and set a regular bedtime routine.

Ultimately, it is important for parents to remain patient and understanding when it comes to bedwetting, as it is a common issue among children that can usually be resolved with the right approach.

Chapter 2

Causes of Bedwetting in Children

1. Urinary Tract Infection: Urinary tract infections (UTIs) are a common cause of bedwetting in children. UTIs occur when bacteria get into the bladder and cause inflammation. Symptoms of a UTI may include pain or burning sensation when urinating, frequent urination, or cloudy or foul-smelling urine.

2. Stress: Stress can contribute to bedwetting in children. This may be due to changes in their environment, such as a new school or home, or due to a traumatic event. Stress can

lead to a decrease in the production of antidiuretic hormone (ADH), which helps the body regulate urine production.

3. Bladder Capacity: Some children may have smaller bladder capacities than others, making it difficult for them to hold in their urine for long periods of time. This can lead to bedwetting during the night.

4. Sleep Disorders: Sleep disorders, such as sleep apnea or restless leg syndrome, can interfere with the body's ability to stay asleep. This can cause the body to wake up more frequently during the night, leading to increased urination and bedwetting.

5. Genetics: Bedwetting is often inherited. If a parent or sibling experienced bedwetting, a

child may be more likely to experience it as well.

6. Medication: Some medications, such as diuretics or antidepressants, can increase the amount of urine produced by the body. This can lead to bedwetting.

7. Underlying Medical Conditions: Some medical conditions, such as diabetes, kidney problems, and neurological issues, can cause bedwetting in children.

Chapter 3

When to Seek Professional Help

If a child is over the age of 5 and has been bedwetting for more than 6 months, it is recommended to seek professional help from a doctor or therapist.

Bedwetting can have physical, emotional, and social effects on a child and can be caused by a variety of factors. A professional can help determine the underlying cause of the bedwetting and provide the appropriate treatment and resources to help the child manage it.

If the bedwetting is causing distress to the child or disruption to the family, it is important to seek help sooner rather than later.

It is also important to note that bedwetting is not a sign of behavioural or emotional problems, and seeking professional help should not be seen as a punishment or source of shame.

It is normal for children to experience bedwetting at some point, and seeking professional help can help the child understand and manage their bedwetting in a healthy way.

Chapter 4

Tips to Help Manage Bedwetting

1. Establish a Bedtime Routine: Establishing a consistent bedtime routine can help prevent bedwetting. Make sure your child is getting enough sleep and has plenty of time to use the bathroom before bed.

2. Limit Fluid Intake: Avoid giving your child fluids close to bedtime. This will reduce the amount of urine produced and reduce the chances of wetting the bed.

3. Use a Bedwetting Alarm: Bedwetting alarms are an effective way to help your

child learn bladder control. The alarm will sound when moisture is detected and helps your child wake up to use the bathroom.

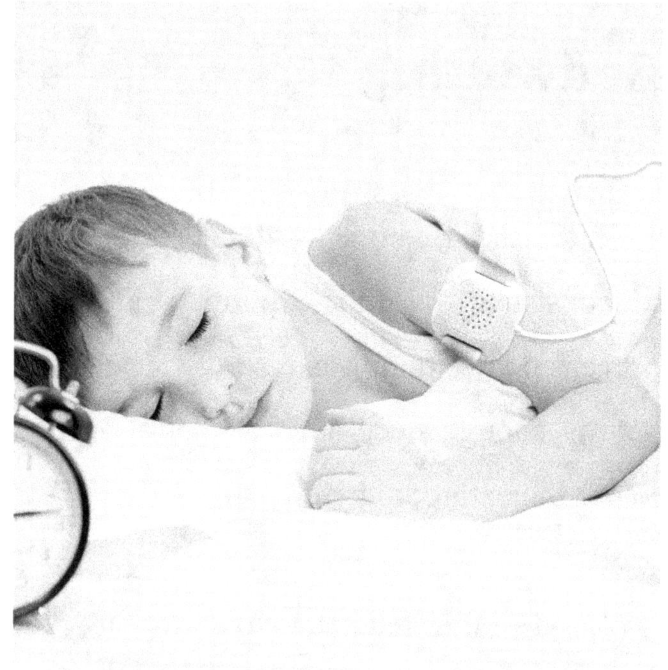

4. Reassure Your Child: Let your child know that bedwetting is a common problem and is nothing to be embarrassed about. Let them know that you understand and can help them manage it.

5. Talk to Your Doctor: If you're concerned about your child's bedwetting, speak to your doctor. They can provide advice and help you find the best solution for your child's situation.

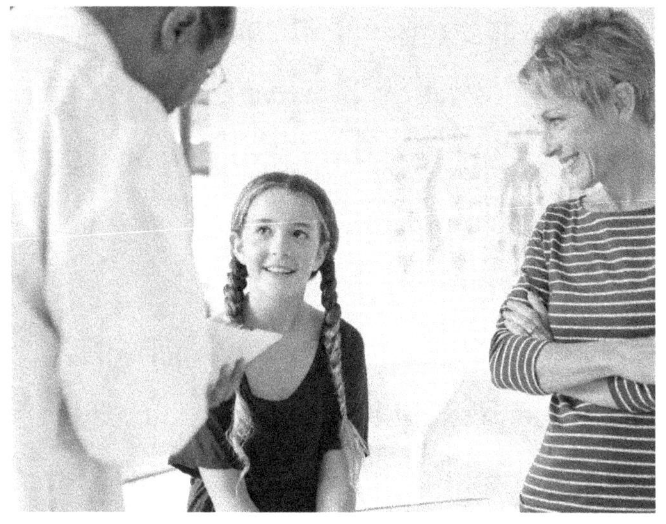

6. Use Nighttime Absorbent Products: Using nighttime absorbent products such as pull-ups or bed pads can help protect the bed and mattress from getting wet.

7. Encourage Your Child to Relax: Make sure your child has a relaxed environment to sleep in. This may include calming music, dim lighting, and a comfortable temperature.

8. Avoid Punishment: Punishing your child for bedwetting is not effective and can be damaging to their self-esteem. Instead, focus on providing support and helping them manage the problem.

9. Keep a Record: Keeping track of your child's bedwetting can help you find patterns and determine the best course of action. Make sure to take note of any changes in behaviour, diet, or environment that may be contributing to the problem.

10. Stay Positive: Bedwetting can be difficult to manage but it can be overcome. Staying positive and encouraging your child will help them stay motivated and continue to make progress.

Chapter 5

Home Remedies for Child Bedwetting

1. Establish a regular toilet routine: Establish a regular toilet routine for your child. Encourage your child to use the bathroom before bedtime and at regular intervals during the day.

2. Set a regular bedtime: Establish a regular bedtime, and stick to it. This will help your child become more aware of the need to go to the bathroom and will reduce the chance of bedwetting.

3. Limit fluids before bed: Try to limit the amount of fluid your child drinks before bedtime. If your child has been drinking a lot before bed, gradually reduce the amount until it is just a few sips.

4. Avoid caffeine: Avoid giving your child any caffeine-containing beverages, such as soda and tea, before bedtime. Caffeine can make it harder for the bladder to hold urine.

5. Try an alarm: A bedwetting alarm is a device that is worn on the child's body and is triggered when the child begins to wet the bed. The alarm will help your child become more aware of the need to use the bathroom and can help reduce bedwetting.

6. Use positive reinforcement: Praise your child for staying dry at night. Offer rewards or incentives to encourage your child to stay dry.

7. Talk to your doctor: If bedwetting continues to be a problem, talk to your doctor about other treatment options. Your doctor may suggest medication or other treatments to help reduce bedwetting.

8. Reduce stress: Try to reduce stress in your child's life as much as possible. Stress can make bedwetting worse.

9. Don't punish your child: Don't punish your child for bedwetting. This can make the problem worse and can damage your relationship with your child.

10. Encourage your child: Let your child know that bedwetting is common and that it is not their fault. Encourage your child to keep trying to stay dry and reassure them that it will get better.

11. Keep bed sheets dry: If your child does wet the bed, make sure to change the bed sheets and mattress right away. This will help keep your child dry and comfortable.

12. Make sure your child is comfortable: Make sure your child is comfortable before bedtime. Make sure the room is not too hot or too cold and that the bedding is comfortable.

13. Use absorbent bedding: Use absorbent bedding, such as mattress pads or waterproof sheets, to help keep the bed dry.

14. Talk to a therapist: If bedwetting is causing your child distress, consider talking to a therapist. A therapist can help your child cope with any anxiety or stress that may be causing the bedwetting.

15. Consider medication: If other treatments don't work, your doctor may suggest medication to help reduce bedwetting.

16. Make sure your child is healthy: Make sure your child is healthy. Certain medical conditions or illnesses can cause bedwetting. If your child is sick or has any medical issues, talk to your doctor.

17. Check for food allergies: Some food allergies can cause bedwetting. If you suspect your child has any food allergies, talk to your doctor about testing for them.

18. Encourage your child to go to the bathroom: Encourage your child to use the bathroom before bed and at regular intervals during the day. This will help your child become more aware of the need to go to the bathroom and can help reduce bedwetting.

19. Consider using a bedwetting alarm: A bedwetting alarm is a device that is worn on the child's body and is triggered when the child begins to wet the bed. The alarm will help your child become more aware of the

need to use the bathroom and can help reduce bedwetting.

20. Talk to other parents: Talk to other parents who have dealt with bedwetting in their children. They may have helpful advice and tips that can help reduce bedwetting in your child.

Chapter 6

Treatment for child Bedwetting

1. Make sure your child is getting the recommended amount of water each day.

2. Have them use the bathroom before they go to bed.

3. Limit their intake of caffeinated beverages.

4. Cut back on any evening snacks.

5. Use positive reinforcement for dry nights.

6. Try using a bedwetting alarm.

7. Help your child relax before bed.

8. Consult with your doctor to rule out any medical issues.

9. Consider using a medication like desmopressin.

10. Talk to a doctor about possible psychological issues.

Conclusion

In conclusion, child bedwetting is a common problem experienced by most children and can be a source of stress for both the child and their parents. However, there are a variety of home remedies that can help to address the issue, including changes to the child's diet and lifestyle, reducing the amount of liquid they drink before bed, and providing supportive measures like bedwetting alarms and rewards systems. With patience and understanding, parents can help their children manage their bedwetting and provide them with the support they need to overcome this issue.

While some children may require further professional help, such as medications or behavioural therapy, these home remedies can be a great first step in the process of addressing bedwetting.

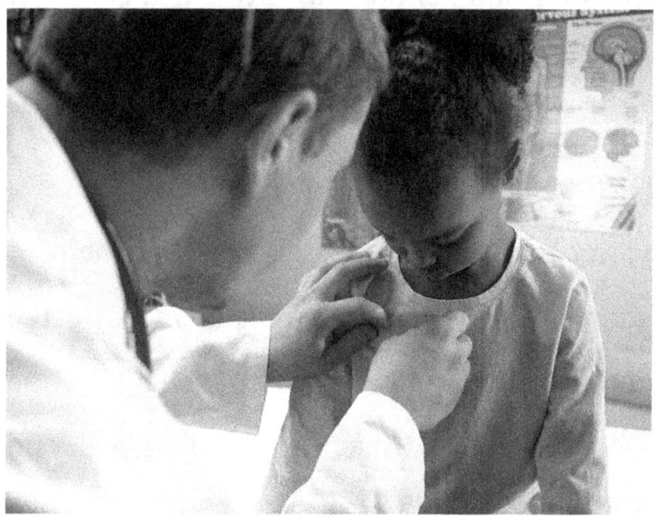

As always, it is important to consult with a doctor before attempting any of these remedies to ensure that they are appropriate for your child.

www.ingramcontent.com/pod-product-compliance
Lightning Source LLC
Chambersburg PA
CBHW050756250726
48662CB00005B/2246